The New Mediterranean Diet Book

A 30-Day Quickstart Guide to
Fast Fat Loss and Amazing
Health (includes Recipes)

JAMES A. PIERCE (CRI)

CONTENTS

Welcome to the Mediterranean Diet!

Are you looking to lose weight and regain your health? There are so many 'diet plans' out there making wild promises of quick weight loss, but there's always a catch, isn't there? Expensive supplements, strange eating schedules, weird food combinations, and unusual eating habits all take their toll. Seriously, kale and Lemon Chicken for breakfast? Who can really live like that long term?

The New Mediterranean Diet is for real people who live normal lives because it's based on real-life eating habits. The traditional diet of the people who live in the Mediterranean region has been scientifically shown to promote healthy weight, health, and longevity. It helps manage and prevent diabetes, heart disease, cancer, and Alzheimer's. It also lets you enjoy real meals, with a glass of wine and some good friends. You can't do that when all you're eating is mangoes for 21 days, can you?

You don't need a Master's degree in biochemistry to understand the Mediterranean diet. You don't have to study the plan and buy special foods before you begin. You can start tomorrow! All you need is a little information, some healthy fresh food in your fridge, and the willingness to make some minor changes to your current eating habits. Really, that's it! There are no withdrawal symptoms, no 'adaptation' period, no eating schedules, and no confusing supplements. Just real food, simply prepared!

The Mediterranean diet is not just a 'diet'. It's a lifestyle, and that means that you can make it a part of your life. You'll be focused on living, not eating, and that means that you can enjoy your meals, your friends, and your family while you regain your health, prevent long-term health problems, and bring your weight back within healthy limits.

In this book, I'll show you how to make the Mediterranean

diet and lifestyle part of your life. You'll learn what to do, why to do it, and how to make it fit seamlessly and easily into your normal daily routine. You can do it all without adding stress to your life or putting a strain on your budget. There's a meal guide to get you started, along with tips for planning your own meals and adapting old family favorites. The recipes you can use to implement the meal plan are also included, as are 'make-ahead' tricks to simplify your meal preparation and your life.

A healthy weight and a healthy life truly are within your reach. The Mediterranean diet can get you there, as well as let you enjoy the journey. Are you ready to take the first step? Then, turn the page!

I: Understanding the Mediterranean Diet

With the incidence of obesity, diabetes, and heart disease rapidly on the rise, many people are looking for a way to lose weight and regain control of their health. There are numerous factors involved in this decline of our health over the past 60 years, and you want a plan that addresses them all. What may be even more important is that you can actually live with the plan, long term. That's the beauty of the Mediterranean Diet!

The Mediterranean Diet is a lifestyle plan more than just a diet. There are no prohibited foods, strange eating schedules or expensive 'special' foods or supplements to buy. It's all about real food, prepared simply. The portions are controlled, and 'healthier' options will fill more of your plate, more often. Other foods are eaten in moderation or in slightly smaller portions than you may have become accustomed to. The Mediterranean Diet is also about balance—not just balancing your food consumption, but also balancing your life. Simple exercise, sharing the preparation of a meal, and taking the time to enjoy eating with friends and family are integral parts of the Mediterranean lifestyle.

While so many fad diets have come and gone over the past few decades, making a big noise and then fading into history, the Mediterranean Diet has calmly and quietly continued to grow in popularity. It's backed by more solid scientific research every year, and it fits easily into our modern lives. Most of the things you'll eat are in your fridge and pantry right now! There's no 'right' way to do it; it can be as individual as you are. You don't need to eliminate any food or food group from your menus; you don't need to fast or feel hungry; you don't need to eat every three hours; you don't need to eat within a limited period of time each day; you don't need to do any of the things involved with the current crop of fad diets.

The Mediterranean Diet is based on thc traditional eating and lifestyle patterns of the people living around the Mediterranean Sea. In the 1970s, when the risk of serious health problems had increased dramatically in Western industrialized countries, researchers led by Ancel Keys looked at health statistics from around the world. They found that the people of the Eastern Mediterranean region lived longer, more disease-free lives than any others, even though the region was poor, war-torn, and had less access to modern medical advances. The research team concluded that the difference must be in their diet and lifestyle. Studying the eating patterns of those people, and comparing them with the Standard American Diet (SAD), gave birth to the 'ideal diet', the Mediterranean Diet.

The difference between the two diets is not so much what is eaten, it's how much of it and how often. Adjusting that, along with reducing the use of saturated fats overall, brings you into the Mediterranean Diet. Interestingly, as areas of the Mediterranean have strayed from their own traditional diets and moved closer to the 'traditional' American diet, the incidence of serious disease has risen dramatically in those areas.

So, what exactly do you eat on the Mediterranean Diet? The base of the food pyramid for this eating plan is vegetables, fruit, legumes, nuts, potatoes, whole grains (like oats and brown rice), whole-grain bread or pasta, fish and seafood, herbs, spices, and extra-virgin olive oil. Poultry, eggs, and dairy products (like cheese and yogurt) are eaten in moderation, and red meat is limited due to its high levels of saturated fats. If you do the grocery shopping for your family, you'll notice that the bulk of the Mediterranean Diet consists of many of the less expensive items that are normally on your list. Eating the MD way is very easy on your food budget!

What do you avoid on the Mediterranean Diet? Just about anything that's 'refined' since that means that parts of the food have been removed, and it has been highly processed. This includes items made with refined grains, such as white bread and regular pasta, and refined oils such as soybean oil, canola oil, and cottonseed oil. Added sugar is also to be avoided, particularly in items such as soda and candy. Fruit is the most common dessert, with small portions of sugary sweets eaten only occasionally.

The Mediterranean Diet is about real food, so anything that's highly processed should be off the table. This includes trans-fats, processed meats like hot dogs and lunchmeat, and anything labeled 'low-fat', 'non-fat' or 'diet', except for low-fat dairy. If it looks like it passed through a factory, it's not healthy 'real' food anymore. If it has chemical additives, hidden added sugar, or artificial flavors or sweeteners, it's not real food anymore. Most of these ingredients bring along their own associated health problems, including throwing your metabolism out of whack so you either gain weight and/or find it extremely difficult to lose any.

Avoiding the abovementioned foods is much harder than you might think. Obviously, the Twinkies will become a once-a-year treat. Many of the other items, however, are hidden in the seemingly 'healthy' things that you buy at the grocery store. You need to learn to read food labels to clear these items off your table and out of your body. Packaged food is tricky, and strange things lurk in unexpected places. Let me give you an example.

I have here a package of instant mashed potatoes. It's one of the top brands, and I picked it up so I could get some mashed potatoes on the table in a hurry when I need to. What might you expect to find in the ingredient list? I use potatoes, milk, butter, and a little salt when I make mashed potatoes, and you probably do the same. Here's what's on the label: potatoes, partially hydrogenated oil, corn syrup solids, salt, maltodextrin, coconut oil, non-fat dry milk, sugar, whey powder...let's stop there, even though there are 6 more ingredients. Do you put sugar in your mashed potatoes? It's the 8th ingredient...but wait, it's actually also the 3rd ingredient (corn syrup solids) and the 5th ingredient (maltodextrin) as well! Three kinds of sugar in mashed potatoes? Whey powder? That's dried protein—but there's already dried milk in there. What's the whey for? Partially hydrogenated oil—I'm not sure what that is, but it's definitely on the 'highly processed' list, right?

I think you see the problem. If I made 'real' mashed potatoes, there would be just four all natural ingredients. The processed product has a lot of sugar and several other things added that I don't want or need in my potatoes. My body doesn't want or need them, either, and their effect on my health, short and long term, can't be good.

Reading labels takes some practice, but learning the common names for added sugar is a good place to start. Sugar gets added to all sorts of things, including toothpaste! If it sounds processed (like 'partially hydrogenated'), stay away from it. Some prepared items will surprise you, pleasantly. My unsweetened applesauce, also from a major national brand, has apples, water, and ascorbic acid. That's the entire ingredient list, just as it should be. [If you're wondering, ascorbic acid keeps the apples from turning dark brown, and home cooks often use citric acid (lemon juice) for the same purpose.]

Start by checking out the things in your pantry. Read the labels on the things you use often. That will point you toward the good brands, like my applesauce, that you want to continue buying, and you'll learn the not-so-good ones, like my potatoes, that you'll want to replace. You'll shop slower when you first start weeding out the overly processed foods, but once you find a good brand your grocery shopping will speed right back up. Enlist the help of your children and spouse to do the label reading on the first couple of trips. If you don't find what you're looking for in the regular aisles, try the organic section. Removing these unnatural additions from your food is key in losing weight, reclaiming your health, and following the Mediterranean Diet.

To quickstart a Mediterranean Diet, here are some quick tips. You'll find more details and specific serving guidelines in the meal-planning chapter.

- Build your meals around vegetables, beans, and healthy whole-grain foods. These should fill about half your plate.
- Use smaller portions of meat and poultry, and eat fish/seafood at least twice a week.
- Have fresh fruit for dessert. Limit portions on sweet desserts to 'just enough' to satisfy the sweet tooth.
- Eat breakfast every day.
- Enjoy a glass of red wine with your dinner.
- Use 'good' fats such as olive oil, nuts, sunflower seeds, olives, and avocado.
- Make sandwiches in a whole-grain wrap, ciabatta, or whole-wheat pita.
- Snack on olives or nuts, or have an apple with almond or peanut butter.
- Switch to whole-wheat pasta or, even better, substitute spaghetti squash or zucchini noodles for pasta.

Make a few lifestyle changes to augment your new Mediterranean Diet as well. Take the time to enjoy your meal. Turn off the TV and engage in conversation while you eat. Get some added exercise every day such as a walk around the block or taking the stairs when you can. These small things can do a lot to reduce your stress levels, and that has an impact on your weight, health, and general well-being as much as what you eat does.

II: Proven Health Benefits of the Mediterranean Diet

The Mediterranean Diet is not a fad. It's been around for a long time—long enough for the health benefits that it offers to have proven themselves over and over. It's more than a 'quick fix'; it's a way of eating and a lifestyle that has been shown in numerous studies to reduce the risks of developing heart disease, cancer, hypertension, type 2 diabetes, Parkinson's disease, and Alzheimer's disease. It has also proven to be successful in healthy weight reduction, and is associated with a lower risk of early death across the board.

Changes in lifestyle in Western countries have escalated in the past 100 years, resulting in an overall unhealthy situation. More and more people work in basically sedentary jobs rather than doing physical work on a daily basis, and they rely on mechanized transportation to get them there. Housewives no longer have to haul and heat the water to wash clothes or wrestle the wet laundry onto and off of an outdoor clothesline. The timesaving conveniences of modern living have been both a blessing and a curse.

Culturally we have not adequately compensated for this reduction of physical labor in our modern lives. The workouts at the gym several times a week do not have the same effect on our bodies, or our health, that regular moderate daily exertion did. Jogging regularly is different from walking to work, walking to school, and walking to the store. Driving your car is nowhere near the same as driving a horse and wagon, in terms of exercise. Gardening is now a hobby, not a necessary daily household chore.

Getting these gentler repetitive types of exercise back into your daily routine is one benefit of the Mediterranean Diet. Integrating moderate exercise into your daily life has been shown to have life-long health benefits. It keeps muscles naturally toned, bones strong, blood circulating well, moods stable, and your metabolism functioning at a slightly elevated level all the time. All of this reduces your risk of developing serious health conditions.

The mechanization of modern life also influenced our eating patterns. Refrigerated trucks made more red meat available year-round and at a lower cost. Airfreight blossomed after World War 2, making that problem worse. We stopped eating 'seasonally' from the fruit of the land. A standard dinner became meat and potatoes, with sweet desserts and snacks daily...and those following the Westernized lifestyle became fatter and sicker every year. Western diets have become laden with fats and sugars; people fill up on meat rather than vegetables or grains; and packaged foods contain all sorts of hidden unnecessary ingredients and potentially dangerous chemical additives.

The Mediterranean Diet turns back the clock on those problems. Eating simple 'real' food with natural nutrients gives the human body the tools it needs to fight disease and repair itself. Lowering the consumption of saturated fats, like those found in red meat and butter, helps to lower cholesterol and reduce the risk of heart disease. Reducing sugar intake regulates blood sugar, helping to prevent and control diabetes. The overall reduction in calories promoted by the portion control aspect of the Mediterranean Diet helps attain and maintain healthy body weight. These all combine to help to reduce your risks of developing other diseases as well.

Any one of these changes can bring you great health benefits, but the Mediterranean Diet combines them to offer you optimal health and longevity. It does all this in an affordable, balanced, and livable manner. With these simple moderate changes to your diet and lifestyle, you can enjoy your life, and a glass of wine with your birthday cake, well into a healthy and active old age.

III: Why Mediterranean Works—The Science

Why do the simple changes in diet and lifestyle found in the Mediterranean Diet promote weight loss and good health? There's not a simple answer to that. Human biochemistry is intricate and complicated, and there are a number of hormones released by our brains that affect everything from our weight to how well we sleep. That said, let's take a look at the science supporting the Mediterranean Diet.

First, the Mediterranean Diet was created to mimic the eating habits of the healthiest and longest-lived people in the world. The health statistics from 22 different countries were used to develop the Mediterranean Diet. Fiber and nutrient-rich vegetables and whole grains, unsaturated fats like olive oil, and unprocessed real food were the key elements promoting good health, good body weight, and longevity. These were amplified by moderate consumption of red wine, moderate daily physical activity, and low stress levels.

In 2014, Dr. David Katz of Yale University's Prevention Research Center was asked to compare the medical evidence for and against all the current mainstream diets. As reported by James Hamblin in The Atlantic (March 24, 2014), here's what Katz had to say:

"The Mediterranean diet, which is additionally defined by high intake of fiber, moderate alcohol and meat intake, antioxidants, and polyphenols, does have favorable effects on heart disease, cancer risk, obesity, metabolic syndrome, and 'is potentially associated with defense against neurodegenerative disease and preservation of cognitive function, reduced inflammation, and defense against asthma.'"

The PREDIMED study involved monitoring over 7000 individuals, some following the Mediterranean Diet and some a control group, for almost 5 years. The results, published in 2013, showed that Mediterranean Diet reduced the risk of stroke by 39%, the risk of diabetes by 52%, and lowered 'bad' cholesterol levels, blood sugar and insulin levels, and blood pressure. Other independent research studies have shown that the Mediterranean Diet reduced the risk of a second heart attack by 72%, helped reverse insulin resistance and metabolic syndrome, and delayed (or prevented) the need for drug-therapy in newly diagnosed diabetics. In many studies, people lost more weight on the Mediterranean Diet than on other diets.

Some specific reasons that the Mediterranean Diet helps produce these sorts of results are as follows:

Type 2 Diabetes: The high fiber from eating more vegetables slows digestion and prevents swings in blood sugar. The low sugar intake also helps to stabilize blood sugar levels.

Heart Disease and Stroke: Refined grains, processed foods, and red meat have all been shown to contribute to cardiovascular problems, as has hard liquor. The Mediterranean Diet replaces these foods with whole grains, fresh food, fish/seafood, and red wine, all of which are better for your cardiovascular system, as well as giving you other health benefits.

Alzheimer's, Parkinson's, and dementia: The high levels of antioxidants on the Mediterranean Diet, combined with improved cholesterol, blood sugar levels, and blood vessel health, all contribute to reducing the risks of developing these diseases.

Longevity: The added natural nutrients from whole grains and other unprocessed foods reduce the risk of a senior becoming frail. Routine moderate physical activity contributes to this effect as well. Also, when you reduce the risk factors for heart disease and cancer, you reduce the risk of death at any age by 20%.

Weight Loss: Several factors of the Mediterranean Diet promote weight loss. Daily moderate exercise and replacing sugars and processed foods with vegetables and natural food are big ones. So is reducing stress. When we're stressed, our brains release a hormone called cortisol, which promotes weight gain and increases the body's resistance to weight loss. Lowering blood sugar and insulin levels also helps to prevent the body from storing fat, and it encourages the body to use existing fat deposits for energy.

IV: Meal Planning and Guidelines

One of the best things about the Mediterranean Diet is the number of options you have for your meals. Whether you prefer eggs, yogurt or cereal for breakfast, Mediterranean's got you covered! There's no one 'right' way to follow the Mediterranean Diet. It's completely customizable to your eating preferences! So rather than give you a day-by-day 'eat this' plan, I'm going to give you the servings guidelines... and a whole lot of suggestions for meals which we've included the recipes for in Chapter 6.

Choose what you like from the menu options, and plan out your week on a sheet of paper. This will not only help you to stay within the recommended servings for the different food groups, but it will also simplify both your meal preparation and your grocery shopping!

I'll discuss that in detail in Chapter 5: Tips, Tricks, & Shopping, and you'll find the recipes in Chapter 6: Eating Mediterranean Style.

The Mediterranean Diet is probably very similar to the way you eat now! The main differences would be switching to olive oil, using exclusively whole-grain products, and replacing red meat with poultry and fish. It's not complicated, and it's not hard. So let's talk meal options, shall we?

Breakfast Options

Breakfast should be eaten daily to kick start your metabolism for the rest of the day, but whether you go heavy or light with it is up to you. Hot cereal, cold cereal, yogurt, smoothies, eggs or pancakes...what's your pleasure? Many breakfast choices are also great for light lunches or dinners, so keep that in mind!

Yogurt or Greek Yogurt

The trick here is to find yogurt without artificial sweeteners or sugar. Read the labels carefully. Choose plain unflavored yogurt that you can flavor yourself, and stick with low-fat. This is often easier to find in the larger containers rather than the individual serving sizes, or try making your own (recipe in Ch. 6). You'll also use some of the plain yogurt in salad dressings and sauces. Take the sharp edge off by adding diced fresh or frozen fruit, nuts, or wheat germ. If you really like it sweeter, get some liquid stevia—a drop or two is all you need. Liquid stevia also comes in a ton of flavors, from chocolate to lemon, which makes a really quick easy way to vary the taste of your yogurt if you eat it often.

Strawberry-Orange Smoothie

Smoothies make a popular on-the-go breakfast, packed with good nutrition. This recipe makes a 20-oz. serving, and you can experiment with variations to your heart's content.

Oatmeal

Full of health benefits, oatmeal also fills you up and sticks by you for most of the morning. Use regular oats, however, and not the instant ones that have been highly processed and are full of sugar. Try making your oatmeal overnight in a crock-pot so it's ready to eat when you wake up!

Breakfast Couscous

Whole-wheat couscous, a Mediterranean and North African staple, makes a terrific hot breakfast cereal with dried fruit and cinnamon.

Cold Cereal

Give your cold cereal a makeover by stirring it into yogurt instead of dousing it with milk. Either way, stick with whole-grain options with no added sugar. Once again, you'll need to read labels with care when choosing cold cereal.

Light Lemon Scones

Bake these delicious light bites ahead of time for a portable breakfast. You can vary the flavor by using other ingredients in place of the lemon, and these scones double as a great dessert as well.

Frittata with Feta

For a heartier breakfast option, weekend brunch or a light lunch/dinner, try a traditional frittata. These are great to make on the weekend and you can use the leftovers for either breakfasts or lunches later in the week. They reheat very well, even in the microwave, and they also freeze well.

Egg Scramble

Potatoes and cheese make this frittata variation both filling and tasty. It's also good as a quick easy meatless dinner.

Fluffy Pancakes

Yogurt in the mix adds the 'fluffy' to these whole-grain

pancakes. Make some and freeze some for quick prep later.

Lunch Possibilities

It's so easy to fall into a rut with lunch, so do some preparation ahead of time. Re-purpose your leftovers to get some relief from the same-old sandwich, and take along some carrots, olives, or cherry tomatoes to munch instead of chips. Try some different types of salads instead of the same bowl of lettuce. Be creative! Keeping meals enjoyable is a big part of the Mediterranean Diet!

Sandwiches

Apart from using whole-grain bread, change up your sandwich by using a whole-wheat wrap or pita, or make some homemade ciabatta rolls. Keep your veggies in a separate bag to add right before eating, so they stay nice and fresh. Use tzatziki or avocado instead of mayo, and throw some olives, sprouts or herbs on there. Avoid processed lunchmeats and instead use sardines, chicken, fish or seafood.

Panini

Once you start making Panini you may never go back to cold sandwiches again! You can make them without buying fancy 'presses', and they reheat with a quick zap in the microwave. In Chapter 6, you'll find two suggestions to get you started making Panini: the Mediterranean Creamy Panini and the Chicken & Roasted Pepper Panini.

'Choose Your Protein' Salad

Meat or fish salads are wonderful tucked into pita bread and they're easy and inexpensive to make. Spice up your tuna, eggs or chicken by adding avocado, olives or capers, along with herbs and spices. Chop in some celery or carrots to give it some crunch, and don't limit yourself to the basics. Sardines, crab, and shrimp are often overlooked when people make this type of salad at home. Whether you eat it by itself, put it in a pita or wrap, or use it on top of greens, protein salads make a hearty lunch.

Greek Salad

A Greek salad is built on tomatoes, cucumbers, and cheese rather than greens. It makes a wonderful change of pace!

Pasta Salad Mediterranean Style

This is a filling vegetarian meal, but you can also add in any proteins you'd like. Play with different shapes of pasta and experiment with using rice or couscous.

Tomato, Mozzarella, & Chickpea Salad

This light lunch can also double as a colorful side dish for dinners. Chickpeas, sometimes known as garbanzo beans, are not only filling but also brimming with protein and healthy fiber.

Quinoa Tabbouleh

Tabbouleh is a traditional salad made with bulgar wheat and sometimes with couscous. This version will introduce you to the wonderful South American grain quinoa, which is very high in protein.

Dinner Suggestions

You have your own favorite dinners, and with a few tweaks you can fit them right into the Mediterranean Diet. The basic rule is to fill half the plate with vegetables, one-quarter with starch, and the remaining quarter is for your protein. If you're focused on weight loss, check the size of your dinner plates. In the 1980s, the standard size for dinner plates increased by 1-1 ½ inches, along with our waistlines! Try to use a 9 ½-10-inch plate—it'll make a difference.

Side Dishes

Artichokes Provencal

Artichokes feature prominently in Mediterranean cooking, and here they make a very different side dish.

Stuffed Tomatoes

This side dish is great with seafood or fish, and it will give you a whole new flavor profile for tomatoes.

Roasted Veggies

Roasting gives some old favorites a brand new taste. Brussels sprouts, broccoli, cauliflower, and mushrooms are popular veggies to pop in the oven, but don't overlook carrots and zucchini either!

Skordalia

This thick potato-garlic sauce makes a great base under fish, but it can double as a sandwich spread or dip as well.

Spicy Cauliflower

With garlic, red pepper, and sesame seeds, this may easily be the best cauliflower you will ever eat.

Main Dishes

Artichokes with Pork Sausage
This makes a beautiful plate, and it's a typical Mediterranean Diet meal in all its simplicity.

Fettuccine with Red Pepper Feta Sauce

The feta cheese sauce makes this recipe a real change from what we think of as 'traditional' pasta sauce.

Shrimp & Pasta

Shrimp, olives, and fresh basil combine for a very quick and easy dinner. Try it with crab or mussels as well.

Vegetarian Lasagna

Going 'meatless' once a week is great for both your health and your budget. This lasagna is hearty, cheesy, and sure to satisfy. Get 'no boil' lasagna noodles that don't require pre-cooking to streamline your dinner preparation.

Sweet & Tangy Chicken

Figs provide the pop of sweetness in this chicken dish, offset by the red wine vinegar.

Seafood Grill

This is a wonderful way to grill fish and vegetables for a quick meal. Although this recipe features halibut, you can substitute cod, flounder or monkfish for a less expensive option.

Lemon Salmon with Limas

This dish, with broiled salmon nestled in a bed of spicy lima beans, will give you all sorts of ideas for new ways to use vegetables.

Greek-Style Salmon Burger

These salmon burgers are brightened up with cucumber and feta. Served alone or on a toasted ciabatta roll, top them with a dollop of tzatziki for a true Mediterranean taste.

Stuffed Salmon

The spinach stuffing makes this salmon dish a nutrition powerhouse. You can use the same technique with many other types of fish.

Grilled Sea Bass

Whole fish done on the grill is a summer favorite in the Mediterranean. Sea bass, red snapper, and striped bass all work equally well in this recipe.

Margherita Pizza (and dough)

This is a classic 'light' pizza, and you can use the dough recipe to create your own favorites.

Dessert Treats

Although fresh fruit often serves as dessert on the Mediterranean Diet, other sweets are not forgotten, just limited. These can range from pudding to cake, and a little square of baklava can really put the bow on a great dinner. The following are some suggestions to get a little Mediterranean into your dessert repertoire.

Biscotti

Crispy, crunchy, and great with coffee, we've all come to love these little twice-baked cookies. They're not hard to make, either, and you can try both the Classic Biscotti and the Wedding Biscotti for two different styles.

Ricotta Cookies

These are light and delicate, just enough after a big meal.

Bocche di Dama

Sometimes called 'the queen of the almond cookies', these have rum-soaked cherries in a light almond dough.

Rice Pudding
A traditional Mediterranean recipe, using basmati rice, this pudding has fruit and spices instead of lots of sugar and milk.

Panna Cotta
This versatile dessert is sort of a cross between custard and gelatin. It's light and refreshing, easy to make, and can be garnished in many different ways.

Ricotta Cake

Lighter than cheesecake, and much easier to make, you'll soon be adding this ricotta cake to your holiday menus on a regular basis.

Tuscan Harvest Cake

This is a traditional part of the grape harvest in Tuscany, and this surprising cake is studded with fresh grapes and lightly dusted with sugar.

V: Tips, Tricks, & Shopping

Top Ten Tips: Use these ideas to help you follow the Mediterranean Diet easily.

1. *Include a vegetable or fruit with every snack and meal.* This is the simple way to make your goal for the day. A handful of raisins can spark up your salad, give you an energy boost, and help to meet your fruit guideline. Apples are a great snack dipped in nut butter of any kind, and don't forget to add lettuce, tomatoes, etc., to your sandwiches!

2. *Know how to divide your plate.* At least half the plate should be fruits and vegetables. That leaves you with one-quarter for your starch and one-quarter for your protein. Simply portioning your servings to meet this guideline will help to boost weight loss and make you feel better, so pile on the veggies!

3. *Make healthy substitutions.* Going with whole grains instead of refined is a start but, to truly lose weight and claim the full benefits of a Mediterranean Diet, take it a step farther. Use vegetable noodles in place of pasta, at least for some meals. They're easy to make, as is spaghetti squash. While brown rice is healthier than white, try some different grains like quinoa and bulgar wheat that pack more nutrition into their calories. You'll add variety to your meals,

boost your nutritional intake, and reduce your calories. Win-win-win!

4. *Use extra-virgin olive oil for everything.* The health benefits of EVOO can't be overstated. In the Mediterranean, it's even used on bread instead of butter (which has animal fats). Use this healthy oil for cooking, seasoning, and dressing whatever you can.

5. *Eat fish and seafood at least twice a week.* Because they are coastal communities, Mediterranean menus feature a lot of fish and seafood dishes. This is one area where modern living has the past beat hands down! You have access to more fresh and/or frozen fish and seafood than ever before. Choose plain options instead of breaded or prepared, and look for sales. Canned versions are even less expensive, and they offer you the same benefits. So make tuna, crab, and shrimp part of your weekly menus.

6. *Eat your veggies first.* One sure way to reduce your calorie consumption and be satisfied with a smaller portion of protein is to fill up on veggies first. Make soup or salad the first course of your meal, even at lunch; then follow it with the main dish and sides. You'll eat more of the healthy stuff, and you'll also find that a palm-sized serving of protein and a fist-sized serving of starch are more than sufficient.

7. *Get physical!* You don't need to train for a marathon or spend hours at the gym. Simple, natural movement is just as beneficial for your health, if not more so. Walk whenever you can. Try stopping by the park on the way home from work, and taking a casual stroll. It will provide more than exercise; you can de-stress and put a buffer between work and home. Use the stairs, park at the far end of the lot, get off the bus a stop early, stand up and stretch once an hour—you've heard all these suggestions before. Start doing some of them and you will improve both your health and your mood. Just get up and move!

8. *Have healthy eating options easily available.* Keep fruit and veggies on hand at home and at work. Pack your own little snacks of fruit, nuts, etc. to keep in your desk and your handbag/briefcase/pocket/car. Get some of those little individual servings of peanut butter to have with an apple. If you have a snack ready and waiting, you're more likely to eat it than to trek to the vending machine for potato chips. Try flavored seltzer waters instead of sodas, or make some strong herbal tea and dilute it with plain carbonated water. Make it easy to snack healthy!

9. *Eat more nuts.* Nuts contain healthy fats and protein, so make them a bigger part of your life. Add them to your yogurt or cereal, drop a handful onto a salad or sprinkle some over your dinner veg. Yes, they are high in calories, so you have to watch the quantity, but the health benefits of nuts can liven up many of your meals.

10. *Laugh more.* Not only does laughing reduce stress, it gives you a physical boost as well. A study at the University of Michigan found that 20 minutes of laughing equaled 3 minutes on a rowing machine in its effect on your lungs and breathing. The Mediterranean Diet is about lifestyle changes as well as food, so lighten up and laugh more!

Tricks: Some suggestions to make your life and food prep easier.

Slow-cookers: Dust it off and simplify your life. You can cook a hot breakfast overnight in the crock-pot, or have tomorrow's dinner already in the crock to pop in first thing in the morning. Make some pulled pork that can serve not just for dinner but also lunch wraps later. Slow cookers can make meal preparation a lot easier, so plan ahead and haul out your crock-pot.

Planned leftovers: Let's face it, leftovers have gotten a bad rap. Many dishes, like lasagna, are even better the second day. Make more than you need for tonight's meal and stash it in the fridge or freezer for quick easy meals later on! Also use pre-cooked chicken from the deli. A whole rotisserie chicken will make a lot of lunches and dinners, and the picked carcass will be a great start for homemade soup. Plan ahead to save time and money on your meals.

Go frozen: There are many fruits and vegetables available 'fresh frozen' in your grocery store's freezer section, without anything added to them. They're economical, healthier than canned, and very easy to keep on hand. But there are other timesaving surprises in the freezer section: pre-diced onions, peppers, and herbs; brown rice and quinoa in microwave steamer bags; baklava and tiramisu in individual-sized servings. Check out what's available and cut your food prep time considerably. It may also give you some good ideas for pre-prepping and freezing on your own.

Buy in bulk or on sale: Use the 'big box' stores to buy larger quantities of things you'll use a lot, such as extra-virgin olive oil. You can funnel it into a smaller bottle for everyday use and still save a lot of money. Fish/seafood and fresh fruits/veggies are also less expensive, so buy large, repackage, and freeze your own. A vacuum sealer is a really handy investment for this. Most supermarkets have online coupons you can load right on to your shopper's card for an automatic discount.

Read the labels: 'All natural', 'organic', and 'heart healthy' are advertising labels that don't mean much when it comes to food. You must look at the ingredient list to see what's really in a food product. Extra and unnecessary salt and sugar are in many things, as are artificial flavors and sweeteners (read as 'chemicals'). Eliminating all these added ingredients will make your meals more flavorful, your waistline smaller, and your overall health better.

Shopping List: Use the following list to guide you, and shop 'the perimeter' of the store where the unprocessed food is. Try to choose the least processed options.

- Vegetables: carrots, onions, broccoli, spinach, cauliflower, garlic, etc.
- Fresh herbs: oregano, basil, mint, dill, etc.
- Fruits: apples, bananas, oranges, grapes, etc.
- Berries: strawberries, blueberries, etc.
- Frozen veggies: Choose mixes with healthy vegetables.
- Grains: whole-grain bread, whole-grain pasta, etc.
- Legumes: lentils, pulses, beans, etc.
- Nuts: almonds, walnuts, cashews, etc.
- Seeds: sunflower seeds, pumpkin seeds, etc.
- Condiments: sea salt, pepper, turmeric, cinnamon, etc.
- Fish: salmon, sardines, cod, trout
- Shrimp and shellfish
- Potatoes and sweet potatoes
- Cheese: feta, fresh mozzarella, etc.
- Greek yogurt, low-fat
- Chicken
- Pastured or Omega-3 enriched eggs
- Olives
- Extra-virgin olive oil

VI: Eating Mediterranean Style

Great sounding meals don't do you a lot of good without the recipes, so here they are for the suggested meals in Chapter 4. Please use these as a starting point for creating both your own menus and for experimenting with new foods and techniques. Your possibilities are endless! Enjoy!

Breakfast Recipes

DIY Yogurt

With a gallon of milk, a slow cooker, a cooking thermometer, and a little 'starter', you can make your own breakfast yogurt right at home. You may find it a little thinner than store-bought because it doesn't have all the added thickeners. It's also missing all the other commercial additives, so it's super healthy! For your starter, you'll need a small container of plain yogurt with live active cultures. Read the label carefully, looking for 'streptococcus thermophiles' and 'lactobacillus bulgaricus'. If the actual bacteria cultures aren't listed, choose a high-quality plain unsweetened organic yogurt. Pick up some cheesecloth for draining, and you're ready to go!

Ingredients: (makes about 20 servings)

- 1 gallon reduced-fat milk
- 2 T. starter yogurt

Directions:

1.   Pour the milk into the slow cooker and heat covered on low setting until it's between 180 and 190 degrees Fahrenheit, as measured on the cooking thermometer. This kills off all bacteria in the milk so the yogurt-creating bacteria can thrive.

2.   Turn off the crock-pot and let the milk cool undisturbed for about 3 ½-4 hours. You want to catch it at 110 degrees Fahrenheit, so check often. If it's too hot or too cold when you add your starter, the bacteria will not do well.

3.   Your milk may develop a 'skin' as it cools, particularly if you use raw milk. Remove this completely or you'll get nasty flakes in your yogurt.

4.   When the milk reaches 110 degrees Fahrenheit, remove about a cup of it. Add your 2 T.

of starter to the milk and gently but completely mix it in with a fork or a whisk. Don't think 'more is better'! Too much starter will inhibit the growth of the good bacteria by overcrowding them.

5.   Add your milk and starter back into the slow cooker. Stir it in very gently, moving slowly from side to side and up and down. Don't whisk it around in circles.

6.   Remove the crock from the base and place it in a cool oven. If you have an electric oven, turn the oven light on; the pilot light in a gas oven will serve also. You want to keep your mixture warm. Tuck a bath towel or winter scarf around your crock, and leave it undisturbed overnight for about 10-12 hours. Don't even open the oven door to peek!

7.   After 10-12 hours, you'll have yogurt in your crock with a layer of whey on the top. Line a colander with three layers of cheesecloth and place it over a large pot. Pour your yogurt into the colander. The whey will drain off down into the pot.

8.   Drain for about 2 hours to get a thick natural yogurt or about 4 hours for Greek style. Lift the cheesecloth from the colander and put the yogurt into a covered storage container.

9.   If you like a sweeter yogurt, store it in the refrigerator immediately after draining. If you like it tart, let it sit out at room temperature for about 24 hours. The longer it sits at room temperature, the

tarter it will get.

10.   Separate out a small amount to use as your starter for the next batch and enjoy!

Strawberry-Orange Smoothie

This makes about a 20-oz. serving that's rich in nutrition. You can add ice to get a thicker texture or use frozen fruit, if you'd like, and definitely try this with different fruits and juices!

Ingredients:

- ½ cup low-fat plain yogurt
- 1 cup of strawberries
- 1 cup orange juice
- 4 T. wheat germ or plain whey protein

Directions:

Put all ingredients in a blender and mix until smooth.

Breakfast Couscous

Couscous is steamed rather than cooked, so this is very quick to prepare in the morning. This recipe makes about four servings.

Ingredients:

- 3 cups low-fat milk
- 1 2-inch cinnamon stick
- 1 cup uncooked whole-wheat couscous
- ½ cup chopped dried apricots
- ¼ dried currants or raisins
- 6 tsp. brown sugar
- ¼ tsp. salt
- 4 tsp. butter, melted

Directions:

1.   Warm the milk and cinnamon stick over medium-high heat in a saucepan about 3 minutes. Heat until small bubbles form around the edges, but do not boil.

2.   Remove the pan from the heat. Add in the couscous, apricots, currants, salt, and 4 tsp. of the brown sugar. Stir well.

3.   Cover and let stand 15 minutes.

4.   Remove and discard the cinnamon stick.

Serve topped with one tsp. melted butter and ½ brown sugar per serving.

on Scones

ᴛ꜇ꜱᴘ.

ᵻic recipe that yields 12 scones. You
lemon zest with lime or orange, or
_ ᵢᵢᵢ dried fruit, nuts, and spices. The
ᴜᴀᴋing aisle of your supermarket has a powdered
buttermilk blend especially made for baking, and
it's easy to keep on hand in your cupboard in place
of liquid buttermilk. If you're interested in weight
loss, skip the frosting step!

Ingredients:

• 2 cups (plus 1/4 cup flour for kneading)
• 2 T. sugar
• 1/2 tsp. baking soda
• 1/2 tsp. salt
• 1/4 cup butter
• zest of one lemon
• 3/4 cup reduced-fat buttermilk
• 1 cup powdered sugar (for frosting)
• 1 to 2 tsp. lemon juice (for frosting)

Directions:

1. Line a baking sheet with parchment and
preheat oven to 400 degrees Fahrenheit.

2. Combine 2 cups of the flour, the sugar, salt,
and baking soda in a bowl or in a food processor.

THE NEW MEDITERRANEAN DIET BOOK

3.   Cut the butter into the mixture until it looks like fine crumbs. If working in a bowl, use a pastry blender or two butter knives to do this.

4.   Stir in the lemon zest and the buttermilk until mixed. Mixture will still be a little lumpy.

5.   Use the remaining flour to cover a flat surface for kneading the dough. Knead gently about six times, folding the flour into the mixture.

6.   Form the dough into a ball then flatten it to about one-half inch thick with a rolling pin.

7.   Cut your dough circle into four pieces then divide each section into three smaller pieces.

8.   Place on baking sheet and bake for 12-15 minutes until golden brown. Cool on a wire rack.

9.   To frost, mix the powdered sugar with the lemon juice, forming a thin liquid that you can drizzle over the cooled scones. You can use water instead of juice for a vanilla drizzle.

Frittata with Feta

An egg dish is a quick easy breakfast, lunch or light dinner, and most people have eggs and cheese in the fridge all the time. Substitute cheeses and veggies to change the taste, and save your leftovers for lunch later in the week. Make this the night before for a quick breakfast in the morning.

Ingredients:

- 8 eggs
- ½ cup low-fat milk
- ½ tsp. salt
- ¼ tsp. freshly ground black pepper
- 1 tomato, diced
- 2 T. fresh chives, chopped
- 2 tsp. olive oil
- 4 oz. feta cheese

Directions:

1.   Preheat oven to 375 degrees Fahrenheit.

2.   Mix eggs, milk, salt, and pepper in a bowl, whisking well. Stir in diced tomato and chives.

3.   In a skillet with an ovenproof handle, heat oil over medium heat. Pour in the egg mixture and top with crumbled feta. Cook 3-4 minutes until it begins to set around the edges.

4.   Place the skillet in the preheated oven, and bake the frittata for 9-10 minutes until the center is set.

Egg Scramble

With potatoes and ricotta, this is a hearty addition to your menu, and it's super quick to get on the table.

Ingredients:

- 1 tsp. olive oil
- 1 tsp. butter
- 3 new potatoes, thinly sliced
- 1/4 large red bell pepper, small diced
- 8 black olives, chopped
- 1/4 cup fresh parsley, chopped
- 1/4 cup fresh ricotta cheese
- 6 eggs
- salt and pepper to taste

Directions:

1.   Heat olive oil and butter in a large fry pan over medium-high heat.

2.   Sauté potatoes for about 15 minutes. Add the bell pepper and olive and cook for an additional 4 minutes.

3.   Whisk together the eggs, parsley, and ricotta in a bowl. Pour into the fry pan, stirring occasionally until eggs are firm and set but not dry. Salt and pepper to taste.

Fluffy Pancakes

This recipe makes 5 servings, so freeze the extras for breakfast later. Serve with light maple syrup and fresh fruit.

Ingredients:

- 1 1/2 cups low-fat yogurt (any flavor)
- 1 egg
- 1 cup whole-wheat or buckwheat pancake mix
- 3/4 cup low-fat milk

Directions:

1. Heat flat griddle or fry pan to medium-high heat.

2. Use about ¼ cup of batter for each pancake, and cook until edges are set and bubbles have formed on surface before flipping.

cipes

a Rolls

Ciab... ia rolls can make your lunch sandwich something special. The 'biga' is the key to that typical ciabatta taste, texture, and crispy crust.

Biga: Dissolve ½ tsp. active dry yeast in ½ cup water. Stir in 1 cup of flour to make a thick paste. Then stir it briskly about 50 times (to build up the gluten). Cover and allow to sit at room temperature for about 8 hours or overnight. It will have big bubbles on the surface and look soupy when ready to use the next day.

Ingredients:

- 2 cups plus 2 T. water
- 1 tsp. active dry yeast
- all the biga
- 4 cups flour
- 2 tsp. salt

Directions:

1. In the bowl of a standing mixer, dissolve the yeast in the water. Scrape in the biga, breaking it into loose pieces. You don't need to dissolve it.

2.   Add the flour and salt and stir into a thick wet dough. Let rest 15-20 minutes so that the flour can absorb the water.

3.   Using the dough hook, knead the dough at medium speed for 15-20 minutes. [Watch that your mixer doesn't 'walk' off the counter!]

4.   About halfway through the kneading time, the dough should begin to form a ball around the dough hook. If it doesn't, increase the speed slightly. Your dough should end up smooth and glossy but still soft.

5.   Cover and let rise, free of drafts, for 2-3 hours until tripled in size.

6.   Dust a work surface heavily with flour. Gently scrape the dough onto the work surface without deflating it. Dust the top with more flour. Use a pizza cutter to cut into 16 pieces.

7.   Move the rolls one at a time to a parchment-covered baking sheet. Press down on rolls to slightly flatten them. Let them rise uncovered for 30-40 minutes.

8.   Preheat oven to 475 degrees Fahrenheit while the rolls are rising. Bake for 20-30 minutes until golden brown. Cool on a wire rack.

Tzatziki

This all-purpose Greek sauce is a great sandwich spread, dip or sauce for meat. The cucumber, dill, lemon, and mint keep the flavor light.

Ingredients:

- 1 cup Greek yogurt
- 1 English cucumber, seeded and finely grated
- 2 cloves garlic, minced
- 1 tsp. lemon zest plus 1 T. lemon juice
- 2 T. fresh dill, chopped
- 1 T. fresh mint, chopped
- salt & pepper

Directions:

1.   In a medium bowl, mix together the yogurt and cucumber.

2.   Add all spices and stir well.

3.   Chill well before serving.

Mediterranean Creamy Panini

You don't need a fancy press to make Panini at home! Use a bacon press or just flatten with your flipper to squash them down. This is a great vegetarian lunch option, using mayo instead of butter to get that crispy golden crust.

Ingredients:

- 1/2 cup mayo made with olive oil
- 1/4 cup chopped fresh basil leaves
- 2 T. finely chopped oil-cured black olives
- 8 slices whole grain bread (1/2-inch thick slices)
- 1 zucchini, thinly sliced
- 4 slices provolone cheese
- 1 jar (7 oz.) roasted red peppers, drained and sliced
- 4 slices crisp bacon

Directions:

1.   Combine ¼ cup of the mayo with the basil and olives in a small bowl. Spread evenly on four bread slices.

2.   Top each slice of bread with zucchini, provolone, peppers, bacon, and the remaining slices of bread.

3.   Spread remaining mayo on the outside of the

bread, and cook over medium heat in a fry pan or on a griddle about 4 minutes per side until cheese is melted and outsides have browned.

Chicken & Roasted Pepper Panini

These are very simple to assemble, especially if you have some chicken already cooked. Use a teakettle filled with water to 'press' your Panini while they're cooking!

Ingredients:

- 1 lb. cooked chicken, sliced about ½ inch thick
- 8 half-inch slices of French, Italian, or sourdough bread
- 8 thick slices fresh mozzarella or fontina cheese
- ½ cup roasted red peppers
- 8 leaves of basil
- 2 T. mayo
- 1 clove garlic, minced
- olive oil

Directions:

1.   Brush one side of each bread slice with olive oil. Mix the mayo and garlic well then spread on the unoiled side of the bread.

2.   On the mayo-side of four slices, layer 1 slice of cheese, 2 T. roasted peppers, 2 basil leaves, chicken, and another slice of cheese. Top with another slice of bread, mayo-side in.

3.   Cook over medium-high heat, under

something heavy, about 5 minutes per side.

Greek Salad

Chockfull of Mediterranean flavor, this great change of pace from green salads.

Ingredients:

- 1 small red onion, halved and thinly sliced
- kosher salt
- 1/4 cup red wine vinegar
- grated zest and juice of 1 lemon
- 1 tsp. honey
- 1 tsp. dried oregano
- freshly ground pepper
- 1/4 cup extra-virgin olive oil, plus more for drizzling
- 12 to 14 small tomatoes, quartered
- 1 cup kalamata olives, halved and pitted
- 5 Persian cucumbers
- 1 4-ounce block Greek feta cheese, packed in brine
- fresh oregano leaves, for topping (optional)

Directions:

1. Put the onion into a bowl of ice water that's heavily salted. Soak for 15 minutes.

2. Thoroughly mix the vinegar, lemon juice and zest, honey, dried oregano, ½ tsp. salt, and ¼ tsp. pepper in a big bowl.

3.   Slowly whisk in the olive oil until well-mixed. Add the tomatoes and olives and toss.

4.   Peel the cucumbers, leaving alternating stripes of peel. Trim the ends. Cut in half lengthwise and then slice into half-inch slices. Mix them in with the tomatoes.

5.   Drain the onion, add it to the bowl, and toss.

6.   Drain the feta and slice into 4 pieces. Divide the salad among four plates, top with feta and fresh oregano, and drizzle with a little olive oil.

Mediterranean Pasta Salad

Peas are terrific for bumping up the nutrition in a cold salad, so keep a bag in the freezer and add them to this and other salads.

Ingredients:

- 8 oz. multigrain pasta
- zest and juice from one lemon
- 2 tsp. olive oil
- 13.5-oz can artichoke hearts in water, drained and chopped
- 8 oz. fresh mozzarella, chopped
- ¼ cup roasted red peppers, chopped
- ¼ cup fresh parsley, chopped
- ½ cup frozen peas

Directions:

1. Cook pasta according to package directions but without added salt.

2. In a large bowl, combine lemon, juice and zest, with 2 T. olive oil and whisk well. Add the artichoke hearts, cheese, red peppers, and parsley. Stir well to combine.

3. Put the peas in the bottom of a colander. Drain the pasta into the colander, but do not rinse. Add the peas and pasta to the bowl and toss to

combine.

4.   Serve warm or room temperature and drizzle with a little more olive oil, if desired.

Quinoa Tabbouleh

Quinoa gives this cold salad a solid protein punch. This is best made the day before, so the flavors have time to 'marry'.

Ingredients:

- ½ cup quinoa, rinsed
- ½ cup lemon juice
- ¼ cup olive oil
- ½ tsp. salt
- black pepper
- pinch of nutmeg
- 3 bunches fresh flat-leaf parsley
- ½ cup finely chopped fresh mint leaves
- 1 pint cherry tomatoes, quartered
- 1 English cucumber, diced
- jarred peppadew peppers or roasted red peppers, chopped finely

Directions:

1. Bring one cup of water to a boil in a saucepan. While waiting, toast the quinoa over medium-high heat in a sauté pan until it smells nutty and starts to pop.

2. Pour the toasted quinoa into the boiling water. Turn heat down and simmer covered until water is absorbed, about 12-15 minutes. Remove

from heat and let cool.

3.   In a small bowl, whisk together the lemon juice, olive oil, salt, pepper, and nutmeg.

4.   In a large bowl, mix the cooled quinoa with the parsley, mint, tomatoes, cucumber, and peppers. Pour the dressing from the small bowl over the salad and toss to mix well.

5.   Let it sit at least 5 minutes before tasting. Add salt and pepper as needed.

Dinner: Side Dish Recipes

Artichokes Provencal

An unusual side dish is always welcome to liven up any dinner!

Ingredients:

- ½ onion, chopped
- 2 cloves garlic, chopped
- 1 T. olive oil
- ½ cup white wine
- 2 tomatoes, chopped
- 2 9-oz packages frozen artichoke hearts
- 1 strip of lemon zest
- ½ tsp. salt
- ½ cup black olives, chopped
- dried basil, salt, & pepper to taste

Directions:

1.   Heat the oil in a skillet. Cook the onion and garlic with a pinch of salt for about 5 minutes.

2.   Add the wine to the skillet and cook until reduced by about half.

3.   Add the tomatoes, the artichoke hearts, 3 T. water, the lemon zest, and ½ tsp. salt.

4. Cook covered for about 6 minutes then stir in the olives. Season to taste with dried basil, salt, and pepper.

Stuffed Tomatoes

To prevent the filling from getting soggy, cook these immediately following preparation. Large summer tomatoes are fantastic done this way!

Ingredients:

- 2 large tomatoes
- ½ cup garlic croutons (packaged)
- ¼ cup crumbled goat cheese
- ¼ cup sliced pitted kalamata olives
- 2 T. reduced-fat Italian salad dressing
- 2 T. fresh thyme or basil, chopped

Directions:

1.   Preheat broiler.

2.   Cut tomatoes in half and push out and discard the seeds. With a knife, cut the pulp out, leaving the tomato skins fairly hollow. Put the tomato halves upside down on a paper towel to drain for about five minutes.

3.   Chop the tomato pulp and place it in a medium bowl. Add all the remaining ingredients. Mix well and fill the tomato shells with the mixture.

4.   Place stuffed tomatoes on a baking sheet or broiler pan. Broil 4-5 inches below the heat for

about 5 minutes. Serve immediately.

Roasted Veggies

This is a quick easy way to make veggies more interesting, especially for kids. Brussells sprouts, broccoli, and cauliflower are terrific done in the oven, and carrots and zucchini take on a 'French fry' appeal. Adjust cook time depending on your chosen vegetables.

Ingredients:

- veggies of choice
- olive oil
- salt

Directions:

1. Clean and cut veggies into bite-sized pieces.

2. Toss veggies in a little olive oil, and then spread on a baking sheet.

3. Sprinkle with salt and bake at 350 until tender, about 20-30 minutes.

Skordalia

This is a thick garlicky potato sauce thickened with sourdough bread. It's great under light entrees such as fish!

Ingredients:

- 1 lb. russet or Yukon gold potatoes, peeled and cubed
- 8 garlic cloves, peeled
- 1 slice sourdough bread, crust removed
- 1/4 cup plain Greek low-fat yogurt
- 4 T. olive oil
- zest and juice from 1 lemon
- 1/2 teaspoon salt

Directions:

1.   Put potatoes in a large saucepan and cover with cold water. Add the garlic cloves and boil for about 15 minutes, until potatoes are fork tender.

2.   Tear the bread into several pieces and put it in a large bowl. Swipe 2-3 T. of water from the potato pot and spoon it over the bread. Stir with a fork until smooth, and then add the yogurt, half the olive oil, and the lemon juice and zest. Stir until you have a smooth paste.

3.   Drain the potatoes and garlic over a large

bowl, keeping the cooking liquid. Add the potatoes to the bread mixture and mash until smooth.

4.   Add in the reserved cooking liquid, about 2 T. at a time, until the consistency resembles loose mashed potatoes. Stir in the remaining olive oil and the salt.

5.   Keep warm until ready to serve.

Spicy Cauliflower

The spicy sauce is made with a little tofu for added protein, and the two kinds of red pepper give this cauliflower its kick. You need two skillets going for this one!

Ingredients:

- 4 tsp. olive oil
- 1/2 large head or 1 small head cauliflower, cut into florets
- salt and fresh ground pepper
- 3 cloves garlic, chopped
- 1 roasted red pepper, seeded and chopped
- 2 T. soft tofu
- 1/2 tsp. crushed red pepper flakes
- 2 T. breadcrumbs
- 1 tsp. sesame seeds

Directions:

1.   In a large pan over medium heat, cook the cauliflower in 3 T. of the oil. Season with salt and pepper, and cook until the cauliflower starts to brown and soften, about 12 minutes. Stir often.

2.   Heat the remaining T. olive oil in a medium skillet, medium-low heat. Sauté the garlic for about 1 minutes; add the roasted red pepper and cook a few minutes more. Transfer to a blender.

3.   Add the tofu with some salt and pepper, and puree until smooth. Add this to the cauliflower, along with the red pepper flakes. Cook for a minute, and then add in the breadcrumbs and sesame seeds. Cook one additional minute before serving.

Dinner: Main Dish Recipes

Artichokes with Pork Sausage

The aromatic cooking broth gives these artichokes their distinctive flavor, and the lemon and sage set off the sausage perfectly.

Ingredients:

- fresh parsley
- 4 cloves garlic
- 2 bay leaves
- ¼ cup dry white wine
- 1 lemon, halved
- salt & pepper
- 8 whole artichokes
- olive oil
- 1 ½ lbs. large sausage, sliced
- 4 fresh sage leaves
- 2 shallots, minced
- 4 cloves garlic, minced
- ½ lemon, cut into paper-thin slices
- ½ chicken stock
- 2 T. butter

Directions:

1.   Bring 2 quarts of water to a boil in a large wide pot. Add the parsley, whole garlic cloves, bay

leaves, wine, and the 2 unsliced lemon halves to the pot. Season with a little salt and pepper.

2.   While the broth is coming to a boil, prepare the artichokes. Wash them under cold water. Remove the outer petals to reveal the soft paler green center ones. Slice about an inch off the top of each artichoke, and trim the stem to reveal the light green underneath.

3.   Place the artichokes into the broth. Cover and simmer over medium-low heat for about 20 minutes, until a knife slides easily into the base. Remove the artichokes from the pot with tongs, and carefully scoop out the 'choke' from the center of each one. Discard the 'chokes'. Carefully split each artichoke in half and set aside.

4.   Using a large deep skillet, cook the sausage in oil until cooked through, about 7-10 minutes. Remove the sausages and set aside.

5.   Add the sage leaves with a little oil to the pan. Cook 2-3 minutes before adding the shallots, minced garlic, and lemon slices. Cook several minutes more.

6.   Add the chicken stock, bring to a simmer, and cook until reduced. Swirl in the butter and a little olive oil.

7.   Return the artichokes and sausage to the pan to warm them, and then serve.

Fettuccine with Red Pepper-Feta Sauce

The sauce in this recipe is a very different 'take' on traditional pasta sauces, and it's sure to delight you. As a new technique, the starchy pasta water is used to dilute the sauce yet keep it sticking nicely to your pasta.

Ingredients:

- 1 lb. whole-wheat fettuccine
- 2 T. olive oil
- 1 onion, chopped
- 3 garlic cloves, peeled and chopped
- 16-oz. jar of roasted red peppers, drained and chopped
- ½ cup chicken or vegetable stock
- 1 cup crumbled feta cheese
- salt & pepper to taste

Directions:

1.   Sauté the onion and garlic over medium-high heat until soft, about 10 minutes. Add the red peppers and cook until they're heated through. Let cool slightly.

2.   Put the contents of the pan into a blender or food processor. Add the stock and all but 2 T. of the feta. Blend until combined, about 30 seconds.

3. Cook pasta according to the packages directions. Save ½ cup of the water when you drain it.

4. Toss the pasta with the sauce from the blender, adding pasta water little by little as needed to thin the sauce while letting it still stick to the pasta.

5. Divide into four servings and top with the remaining feta.

Shrimp & Pasta

This is a quick, easy, and colorful dinner that's fine with either fresh or frozen shrimp. Try it with crab as well!

Ingredients:

- 2 tsp. olive oil
- 2 garlic cloves, minced
- 1 pound medium shrimp, peeled and deveined
- 2 cups chopped plum tomatoes
- 1/4 cup thinly sliced fresh basil
- 1/3 cup chopped pitted kalamata olives
- 2 T. capers, drained
- 1/4 teaspoon freshly ground black pepper
- 8 oz. whole-wheat angel hair pasta
- 1/4 cup crumbled feta cheese

Directions:

1. Cook pasta following the directions on the package.

2. In a large skillet, heat the oil over medium-high heat. Sauté the garlic for about 30 seconds. Add the shrimp for about a minute, and then the tomato and basil.

3. Reduce the heat and simmer until tomatoes are tender. Stir in the olives, capers, and black

pepper.

4.   Combine shrimp and pasta in a large bowl, tossing well. Top with the feta.

Vegetarian Lasagna

Mushrooms give this vegetarian dish a meaty texture and the zucchini keeps it light. Like many other lasagnas, this is almost better the next day.

Ingredients:

- 2 T. olive oil
- 2 cups mushrooms, sliced
- 6 cloves garlic, chopped
- 2 (14.5-oz.) cans no-salt-added diced tomatoes
- 1 tsp. teaspoon dried oregano
- 6 oz. baby spinach
- 8 oz. low-fat cottage cheese
- 2 medium zucchini, cut lengthwise into 1/4-inch slices
- 1/2 tsp. salt
- 9 no-boil lasagna noodles
- 2 cups shredded low-fat mozzarella cheese

Directions:

1.   Preheat oven to 350 degrees Fahrenheit. Prepare an 8x12 glass baking pan by drizzling 1 T. of olive oil in the bottom.

2.   Heat the remaining olive oil in a fry pan over medium heat. Cook the mushrooms for 5 minutes, and then add the half the garlic, the tomatoes, and ½ tsp. oregano. Let simmer for about 6 minutes.

3.   Microwave the spinach with 2 T. of water for about 2 minutes. Drain and squeeze to remove excess liquid. Mix it with the cottage cheese and the remaining garlic and oregano.

4.   Lay the zucchini slices across the width of the baking dish. Sprinkle with salt. Top with lasagna noodles.

5.   Spread the spinach-cheese mixture in the pan as the next layer and top with more lasagna noodles.

6.   Pour about half of the tomato sauce on top, spreading evenly. Cover with the remaining noodles. Top with the rest of the sauce, making sure all the noodles are covered. Sprinkle with cheese.

7.   Cover with foil and bake for about 35 minutes. Remove the foil and return to the oven until brown and bubbly on top.

8.   Allow to sit a few minutes before trying to slice and serve.

t & Tangy Chicken

s an interesting and unusual mixture of Mediterranean flavors that's served over arugula instead of pasta.

Ingredients:

- 2 tsp. olive oil
- 8 small skinless chicken thighs
- 1/4 tsp. salt
- 2 garlic cloves, minced
- 1/2 c. chicken stock
- 1/4 c. red wine vinegar
- 2 tsp. cornstarch
- 2 tsp. brown sugar
- 3/4 c. Mission figs
- 1/4 c. salad olives
- 1 bag baby arugula

Directions:

1.   Heat oil in a large fry pan over medium-high heat until very hot. Add the chicken, sprinkle with salt, and cook 17-20 minutes until chicken is browned and cooked through. Remove chicken from pan and set aside.

2.   Add the garlic to the pan and cook about 30 seconds. In a small bowl, whisk together the stock, vinegar, cornstarch, and sugar. Add to the pan and

bring to a boil. Continue to boil until the pan is deglazed and the sauce thickens.

3. Stir in the figs and olives, and add the chicken (and any juices) back in. Make sure the chicken is nicely warm again.

4. Serve by spooning over arugula on a plate.

Seafood Grill

Using a grill pan ensures more consistent heat than cooking on an outdoor grill, but either way you'll enjoy this grilled combination of fish and veggies.

Ingredients:

- 1 lb. halibut, cut into 4 pieces
- ½ tsp. salt
- ¼ tsp. dried thyme
- 2 red bell peppers, quartered
- 1 lb. zucchini, diagonally sliced into 1-inch pieces
- ½ red onion, sliced
- olive oil

Directions:

1.   Preheat a grill pan over medium-high heat.

2.   Drizzle olive oil over the fish and sprinkle with salt and thyme.

3.   Grill the fish 2-3 minutes per side. Remove fish from the grill, cover, and keep it warm until serving.

4.   Place the veggies in a bowl and drizzle with olive oil, tossing to coat. Put the bell peppers on the

grill and cook for about 5 minutes. Add on the remaining veggies and continue cooking for about 10 minutes, until veggies are tender, turning as necessary.

Lemon Salmon with Limas

Putting your protein on a bed of beans or other vegetables, instead of a starch, is a great way to raise the nutrition level of your meals. Try this with any kind of beans or get adventurous and use some veggie noodles. The starch saving allows you to have some hot crusty bread with your meal!

Ingredients:

- 1 lemon, halved
- 1/2 cup non-fat plain Greek yogurt
- 3/4 tsp. paprika
- 2 tsp. extra-virgin olive oil
- 3 cloves garlic, thinly sliced
- 3/4 tsp. dried oregano
- pinch of red pepper flakes
- 1 lb. frozen baby lima beans
- kosher salt and freshly ground pepper
- 2 T. fresh parsley, chopped
- 4 skinless center-cut salmon fillets

Directions:

1. Cut one half of the lemon into 4 thin slices. Grate the zest from the other half of the lemon. Set both aside. Preheat the broiler.

2. Squeeze the juice from the zested lemon into a bowl. Add the yogurt and ¼ tsp. paprika. Stir

well.

3.   In a medium saucepan, heat about a teaspoon of olive oil. Add the garlic, oregano, and red pepper flakes. Cook until the garlic has softened. Add the lima beans, the lemon zest, and about 1-½ cups of water. Bring to a simmer, and cook partially covered for about 20 minutes until the limas are tender.

4.   Season the beans with salt and pepper. Remove the saucepan from the heat. Stir in the parsley, 1 teaspoon of olive oil, and 1 tablespoon of the yogurt mix.

5.   Mix ½ teaspoon of salt with ½ teaspoon paprika and a little black pepper, and use this to sprinkle over the fish fillets.

6.   Arrange the fish on a foil-lined baking sheet or broiler pan and put a lemon slice on top of each one. Broil until cooked through, about 6-8 minutes.

7.   Serve on a bed of the lima beans, topped with some of the remaining yogurt mixture.

Greek-Style Salmon Burger

You can make this with canned salmon to save some time, and these burgers are great on toasted ciabatta rolls! Also, try them with tuna and cheddar instead.

Ingredients:

- 1 pound skinless salmon fillets, cut into 2-inch pieces
- 1/2 cup panko
- 1 large egg white
- 1 pinch kosher salt
- 1/4 tsp. freshly ground black pepper
- 1/2 cup cucumber slices
- 1/4 cup crumbled feta cheese
- tzatziki

Directions:

1.   Put the salmon, panko, and egg white into the bowl of a food processor. Pulse until finely chopped. (If using canned salmon, mix these three ingredients by hand in a bowl.)

2.   Form the mixture into 4 patties, and season them with salt and pepper.

3.   Cook on medium-high heat, turning once, for about 5-7 minutes per side.

4. Serve on a bun and topped with the cucumber, feta, and a dollop of tzatziki.

Stuffed Salmon

Here's another technique for cooking fish that you can adapt for different varieties. These thin fillets are rolled around a filling and baked, for an easy-to-prepare main dish.

Ingredients:

- 2 T. olive oil, divided
- 16 oz. frozen spinach, thawed and drained
- 2 T. crumbled feta cheese
- 1 tsp. dried mint
- salt& pepper to taste
- 4 salmon fillets, skinned
- 2 cups vegetable broth
- juice from 1 lemon

Directions:

1.   Preheat oven to 350 degrees Fahrenheit. Grease bottom of a deep baking dish with 1 T. olive oil.

2.   Over medium heat, cook spinach in 1 T. olive oil for about a minute. Add the salt, pepper, mint, and feta. Stir just to combine and remove from the heat.

3.   Spread about ½ cup of spinach mixture on top of each salmon fillet. Roll up the fillet and place

in the baking dish. Turn once to coat with olive oil. Pour the vegetable broth into the dish, and pour the lemon juice over the salmon.

4.   Cover with foil and bake for about 20 minutes until fish is cooked through.

Grilled Sea Bass

Grilled whole and filleted at the table, sea bass makes a tremendous summer meal.

Ingredients:

- 2 lemons
- 3 T. olive oil
- 1 T. fresh oregano, chopped
- 1 tsp. ground coriander
- 1 ¼ tsp. salt
- 2 whole sea bass
- ¼ tsp. black pepper
- 2 large oregano sprigs

Directions:

1. Prepare a charcoal or gas grill for covered cooking over medium heat.

2. From one of the lemons, grate 1 T. of zest and squeeze 2 T. of juice. The remaining lemon should be cut into slices (half) and wedges (half).

3. Mix the olive oil, lemon juice, zest, chopped oregano, coriander, and ¼ tsp. salt in a small bowl. Set aside.

4. Rinse the sea bass and pat them dry. Sprinkle them inside and out with pepper and the

remaining salt. On each fish, make three cuts into the body on each side. Put the lemon slices and sprigs of oregano inside the cavity of each fish, and put the fish into a glass baking dish. Rub half of the oil mixture over the outside of each fish. (Save the remaining oil mix.) Let the fish stand at room temperature for about 15 minutes.

5.   Grease the rack of the grill and put your fish on the preheated rack. Cover the grill, and cook for 12-14 minutes, turning once.

6.   To serve, run a knife along the backbone of each fish, lifting off the top fillet. Remove backbone and rib bones and discard. Drizzle fillets with the remaining oil mix and serve with lemon wedges.

Margherita Pizza (and dough)

Light on the sauce and easy on the cheese, this Italian-style pizza is also easy on your waistline. The dough, the fresh tomatoes, and the fresh mozzarella are the stars of this dish.

Dough:

- 1 ¼-oz package active dry yeast
- 2 tsp. honey
- 1-1/4 cups warm water
- 2 T. olive oil
- 1 tsp. sea salt
- 3 cups flour

Directions:

1.   In the bowl of a stand mixer or food processor, combine the yeast, honey, and warm water. Let 'proof' for 5 minutes. Attach dough hook.

2.   Add the olive oil and salt and mix for 30 seconds. Slowly add the flour ½ cup at a time, mixing for a couple of minutes between additions.

3.   Let the mixer knead the dough for about 10 minutes, adding a little extra flour if it starts to stick.

4.   Remove the dough and let it rest under a

warm, slightly moist towel for about 15 minutes.

Pizza:

- 1 batch pizza dough
- ¼ cup flour
- 2 T. olive oil
- ½ cup crushed canned tomatoes
- 3 plum or Roma tomatoes, sliced in ¼ inch pieces
- ½ tsp. sea salt
- 6 oz. fresh mozzarella, sliced ¼ inch thick.
- ½ cup fresh basil, rough chopped

Directions:

1. Preheat oven to 450 degrees Fahrenheit.

2. Roll the pizza dough out to ½ inch thickness, sprinkling with flour as needed. Prick the dough all over with a fork and put it on a baking sheet. Bake for 5 minutes and then remove it from the oven.

3. Drizzle the crust with the crushed tomatoes and the oil. Place the tomato slices on the crust and sprinkle with salt. Blot the mozzarella slices with a paper towel and place them on the pizza. Sprinkle the whole pie with the basil.

4. Bake for another 15 minutes until cheese is bubbly. (If you want to brown the cheese, pop the

pizza under the broiler for 2-3 minutes.) Let cool a few minutes before slicing.

Dessert Recipes

Classic Biscotti

These are simple and traditional biscotti with the classic anise flavoring. You can easily change the flavoring extract for an enormous variety of flavors.

Ingredients:

- ½ cup vegetable oil
- 3 eggs
- 1 cup sugar
- 1 T. anise extract
- 3-1/4 cups flour
- 1 T. baking powder

Directions:

1.   Preheat oven to 375 degrees Fahrenheit, and line 2 baking sheets with parchment.

2.   Beat together oil, eggs, sugar, and flavoring in a medium bowl until well blended.

3.   In a separate bowl (or large sifter) mix the flour and baking powder well. Add this to the egg mixture, blending in well. You will have a heavy dough.

4.   Divide dough into 2 pieces. Roll each piece into a log the length of your baking sheet. Place each roll onto a baking sheet, and flatten it with your hand to about ½-inch thick.

5.   Bake 25-30 minutes until lightly browned. Remove to a wire rack to cool.

6.   When the rolls are cool enough to handle, cut each roll crosswise into slices about ½-inch thick. Place each slice cut-side up back onto the cookie sheets. It should be lying flat.

7.   Return the biscotti to the oven for about 6-8 minutes. Flip each one and bake the other side for 6-8 minutes. The pieces should be slightly toasted on each side. Place on wire rack to cool.

Wedding Biscotti

Mediterranean cooking uses herbs in baking more frequently than other areas. The fresh rosemary and the currants give these biscotti a very unique taste.

Ingredients:

- 3-1/2 cups flour
- 1 T. baking powder
- ½ tsp. salt
- 2-1/2 T. fresh rosemary, very finely chopped
- 1 stick of butter
- ¾ cup sugar
- 3 eggs
- 1 tsp. vanilla extract
- ¾ cup dried currants

Directions:

1.   Preheat oven to 350 degrees Fahrenheit.

2.   In a medium bowl, mix together the flour, baking powder, salt, and rosemary. Set aside.

3.   In the large bowl of a mixer, beat the butter and sugar together until fluffy, about 4 minutes. Add the eggs one at a time, beating fully between each addition. Mix in the vanilla.

4.   Stir the flour mixture into the egg mix until combined. Add in the currants and stir well.

5.   Divide the dough and shape it into 2 logs, each about 1-inch thick. Bake for about 35 minutes until the edges begin to brown. Remove from oven and let cool on the baking sheets.

6.   While still warm, cut each log on the diagonal into ½-inch slices. Place the slices back on the baking sheets, cut-side up. Bake for 7-8 minutes, flip the biscotti, and cook for another 7-8 minutes.

7.   Let cool a few minutes on the baking sheets before removing to wire rack.

8.   Store (when completely cooled) in an airtight container for up to 2 weeks.

Ricotta Cookies

These are small and light, with just a hint of 'cheesecake' flavor. You can drizzle on a little frosting or sprinkle with colored sugar while they're hot for added sweetness.

Ingredients:

- 2 cups sugar
- 1 cup butter, softened
- 15-oz low-fat ricotta cheese
- 2 tsp. vanilla extract
- 2 eggs
- 4 cups flour
- 2 tsp. baking powder
- 1 tsp. salt
- 1-1/2 cups confectioner's sugar (for frosting)
- 3 T. milk (for frosting)

Directions:

1.   Preheat oven to 350 degrees Fahrenheit.

2.   In large mixer bowl, cream together the sugar and butter at low speed until blended. Increase to high speed and beat about 5 minutes until fluffy.

3.   Reduce to medium speed and beat in the ricotta, vanilla, and eggs, mixing well.

4.   Reduce speed to low and add the flour, baking powder, and salt. Mix until dough forms.

5.   Using a level teaspoon, drop dough onto ungreased baking sheets. Cookies should be small.

6.   Bake at 350 degrees Fahrenheit until slightly browned, about 15 minutes. Let cookies sit a few minutes before removing them to a wire rack to cool. They will be soft, not crisp.

7.   When cooled, mix frosting ingredients and drizzle frosting over the cookies and allow about an hour for the icing to dry completely before storing.

Bocche di Dama

Bocche di Dama, sometimes translated as 'Lady's Kisses', is a delectable sweet morsel to end a meal, almost a marzipan. While this recipe uses cherries soaked in rum, you can substitute other fruit and even nuts, soaked in liqueurs or flavoring extracts. Although not 'traditional', chocolate-coated hazelnuts would be fantastic! Get creative with these! Dragees can be purchased at craft stores that have a baking section, as can mini baking cups.

Ingredients:

- 1 lb. almonds, peeled and very finely chopped
- ½ lb. sugar
- zest from 2 lemons
- 3 egg whites
- wild or sour cherries, soaked in rum for 30 minutes
- mini silver dragees (for decorating)
- mini baking cups
- ¾ lb. confectioner's sugar (for icing)
- ¾ cup milk (for icing)

Directions:

1. If you need to prepare the almonds, boil them to remove the skins easily. Once they are cooled and dry, use a food processor or blender to chop them up very fine.

2.   Preheat oven to 375 degrees Fahrenheit.

3.   In a large bowl, mix the almonds, lemon zest, sugar, and egg whites. It will become a paste-like consistency.

4.   Roll a clump of the paste into a ball about the size of a golf ball. Press an opening into with your finger and put 1-2 cherries inside, depending on the size of the cherries. Roll the dough closed around the filling. Place each one on a cookie sheet.

5.   Bake for about 30 minutes and then let them cool.

6.   Mix the icing ingredients into a thick liquid. Use a basting brush to ice the top of each cookie. Place mini dragee (a little silver ball) or a small piece of dried fruit or nut on top immediately, while the icing is wet. Put each cookie into a mini baking cup.

7.   Let the icing set for several hours (to dry well) before storing.

Rice Pudding

A simple easy dessert, Mediterranean-style rice pudding is lighter than other versions. Try it with the rose water, if you can find it!

Ingredients:

- 1/2 cup basmati rice
- 4 cups milk
- 3 T. sugar
- 1/4 cup raisins
- 1/2 tsp. cardamom
- 1/4 tsp. cinnamon
- 1/2 tsp. rose water (optional)
- 1/4 cup almonds, chopped (garnish)
- 1 T. orange zest (garnish)

Directions:

1.   Soak the rice for 10 minutes in water. Drain well.

2.   Put the milk and sugar into a heavy saucepan. Bring them to a slow boil over medium-high heat.

3.   Reduce heat and add the rice, raisins, cardamom, and cinnamon. Simmer over low heat, stirring frequently, for about 45 minutes until thickened.

4.   Remove from heat and stir in the rose water.

5.   Combine the almonds and orange zest. Divide pudding into 6 servings and garnish with the nut mixture. Serve warm or cold.

Panna Cotta

Panna Cotta is a creamy gelatin dessert that can be garnished with anything you'd like. A sauce, such as caramel or chocolate, can be drizzled right into the bottom of the mold, or you can top the panna cotta off with fresh or frozen fruit. Either way, it's a very light and delicious make-ahead dessert.

Ingredients:

- 1 tsp. unflavored gelatin
- ¾ cup plus 2 T. heavy whipping cream
- 3 T. whole milk
- 2 T. sugar
- 2 T. honey
- 1 cup berries

Directions:

1. Prepare custard cups or individual molds with very light coating of cooking spray. This makes it much easier to get the dessert out of the molds in one piece later!

2. Place ¼ cup of the cream in a small bowl and sprinkle the gelatin into it. Allow it to stand for a minute so the gelatin will soften.

3. Use a heavy saucepan to heat the remaining cream, the milk, and the sugar over medium heat.

Bring to a boil, stirring continuously to prevent scorching.

4.   Remove the cream mixture from the heat once it boils. Stir in the cream and gelatin mixture until it dissolves.

5.   Pour into 4 custard cups or molds, dividing evenly. Chill for at least 4 hours.

6.   To serve, unmold each serving onto an individual serving plate/dessert bowl. Drizzle with a little honey and add the berries.

Ricotta Cake

Rich and citrusy, this cake is very easy to make, and it's a classic Italian dessert that's sure to delight. It's baked at two different temperatures, so watch your timer!

Ingredients:

- 3 lbs. fresh ricotta cheese
- 8 eggs
- ½ lb. sugar
- zest from one lemon
- zest from one orange
- butter (to prep the pan)

Directions:

1. Preheat oven to 425 degrees Fahrenheit.

2. Grease the sides and bottom of a 9-inch spring-form pan generously with butter.

3. Mix all ingredients together in a large bowl and pour into the pan.

4. Bake for 30 minutes. Reduce oven temperature to 375 degrees Fahrenheit and continue baking for an additional 40 minutes.

5. Let cool completely, open up the spring-form

pan, and serve.

Tuscan Harvest Cake

A typically 'low-rise' Mediterranean cake, the combination of fresh grapes and almonds makes this not only a delicious dessert but also very unusual one.

Ingredients:

- ¾ cup flour
- ½ cup ground almonds
- ½ cup corn meal
- 2 tsp. baking powder
- ½ tsp. salt
- 1/3 cup vegetable oil
- ¾ cup light brown sugar
- 1 tsp. almond extract
- 3 eggs
- ½ cup sour cream
- 2 cups red seedless grapes
- 1 T. white sugar
- 1 T. dark brown sugar

Directions:

1.   Preheat oven to 350 degrees Fahrenheit and grease the inside and bottom of a 9-inch spring-form pan.

2.   In a small bowl, combine the flour, ground almonds, corn meal, baking powder, and salt.

3. In a large bowl, combine the oil, brown sugar, and almond extract. Add the eggs one at a time, mixing well after each addition. Stir in the sour cream.

4. Add the flour mixture to the wet ingredients. Stir to mix well. Pour into the pan.

5. Bake for 10 minutes. Remove from oven, and evenly spread the grapes over the top of the cake. Mix the white and dark brown sugars together and sprinkle on top the cake over the grapes.

6. Return the cake to the oven (@350 still) and bake for another 30-35 minutes.

7. Let cool completely before removing from the pan.

Final Thoughts on Living the Mediterranean Lifestyle

Finding a reasonable and effective plan to help you lose weight and improve your health should not be a daunting task. Current 'healthy' diet plans are complicated, expensive, and sometimes downright weird. But, you don't have to struggle with all that. Really, you don't! The Mediterranean Diet offers you the means to reach your goals, without a major upheaval in your life or a major dent in your pocketbook.

By making the slight changes to your lifestyle and diet that have been discussed in this book, you can quickly begin to turn things around. Pounds and inches will start to melt away, and you'll feel better and have more energy. The Mediterranean Diet is easy to follow both now and for the rest of your life. By doing so, you'll reduce your risk for heart disease, Type 2 diabetes, high blood pressure, Alzheimer's disease, obesity, and even cancer. You'll increase your chances of having a long healthy retirement, free from long-term medications and complications. That's a precious gift, to your family and to yourself.

Don't wait. Start modifying your meals today, and start looking better and feeling healthier! Eliminate the sugar and processed foods that are dragging you down, leave the fad diets behind, and get back to eating real food, simply prepared. Come home to the Mediterranean Diet for good taste and good health.